# Life With J.A.K
# LIVING WITH ALBINISM

**Inspired by Julian Aric Kidd, Jr.
Written by Tikia Kidd**

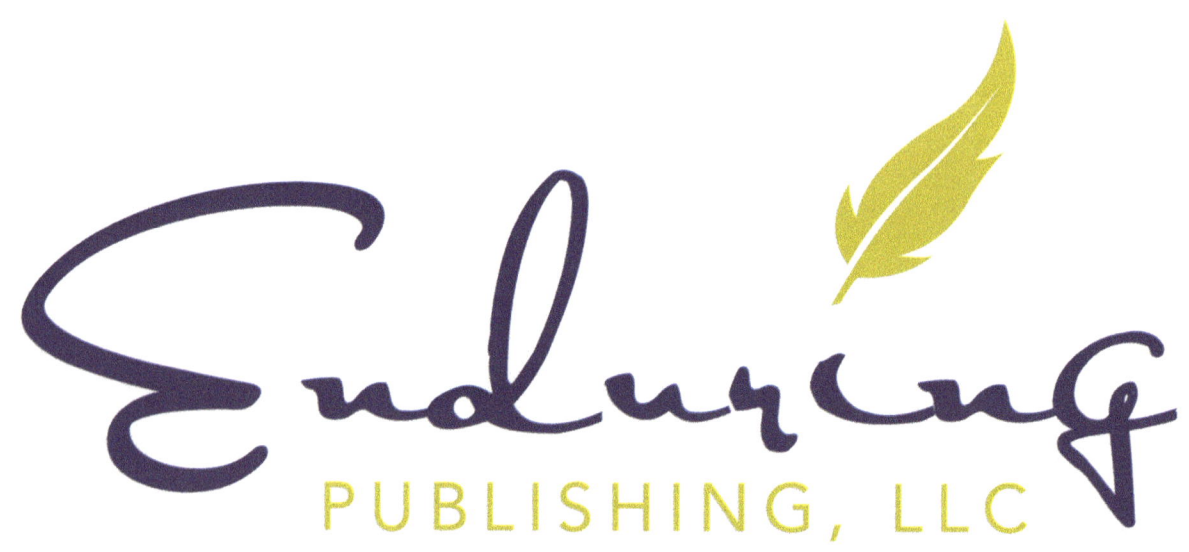

Copyright © 2019 by Tikia Kidd

All rights reserved. No part of this publication ma be reproduced, stored in a retrieval system, or transmitted in any form or by any means - electronic, mechanical, photocopy, recording, or any other - except for brief quotations in printed reviews, without prior permission of the publisher.
Book Design by Enduring Publishing, LLC

**ISBN: 978-0-9971719-0-7**

Printed in the United States of America

First Printing, 2019

*This book is dedicated to my children, who bring me joy, laughter, and love daily, Korryn A. Kidd, and Julian A. Kidd Jr.*

*For all the children who are different. Guess what? All human beings are different. YOU were created to be better than normal.*

*A special thank you to the BEST husband ever!!!*

*Thank you to Enduring Publishing, LLC*

*Love, Kia*

# TABLE OF CONTENTS

1
**Person With Albinism (PWA)**
3
**What Is Albinism?**
4
**How Did I Get This Condition?**
6
**How Do I Protect My Skin?**
10
**Why Do My Eyes Move?**
12
**My Team-Up**
14
**How School Works for Me**
16
**NOAH**
21
I Love Me

# Person With Albinism (PWA)

Hi, my name is Julian A. Kidd, Jr., also known as "JAK" because of my initials. I am four years-old and I have a skin condition called Albinism.

# This is me!

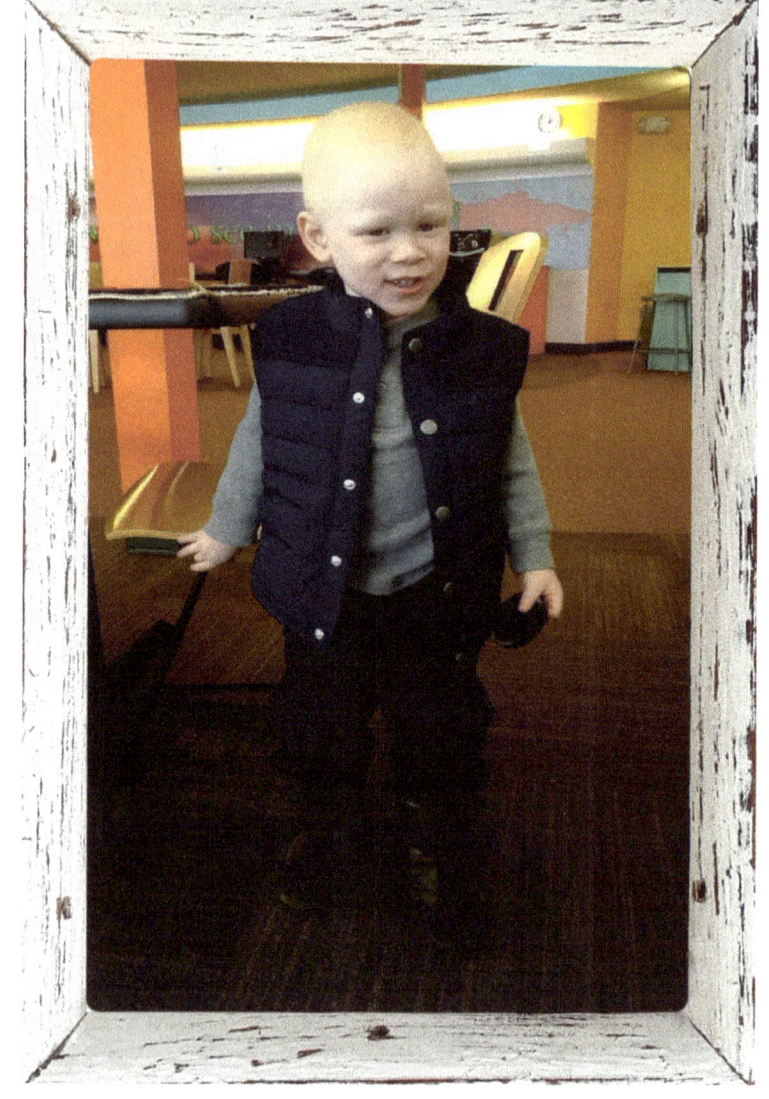

# What Is Albinism?

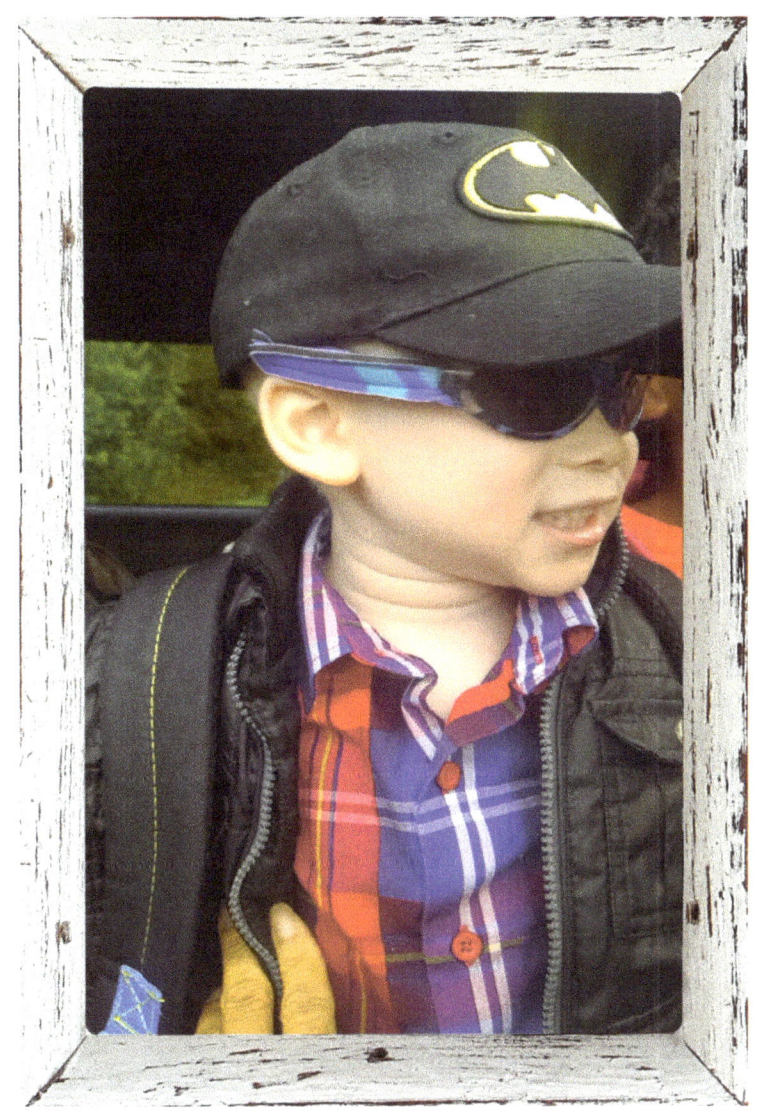

Albinism is a genetic condition that affects the color of my skin, my hair, and my eyes. It also makes seeing far away challenging, but I manage.

# How did I get this condition?

Both of my parents carry the Albinism gene and that is the only way I could have been born with Albinism. The Albinism gene is sort of like the "Clark Kent" of genes.

*Genes play an important role in determining physical traits — how we look —and lots of other stuff about us. They carry information that makes you who you are and what you look like: curly or straight hair, long or short legs, even how you might smile or laugh. Many of these things are passed from one generation to the next in a family by genes. Source: https://kidshealth.org/en/kids/what-is-gene.html

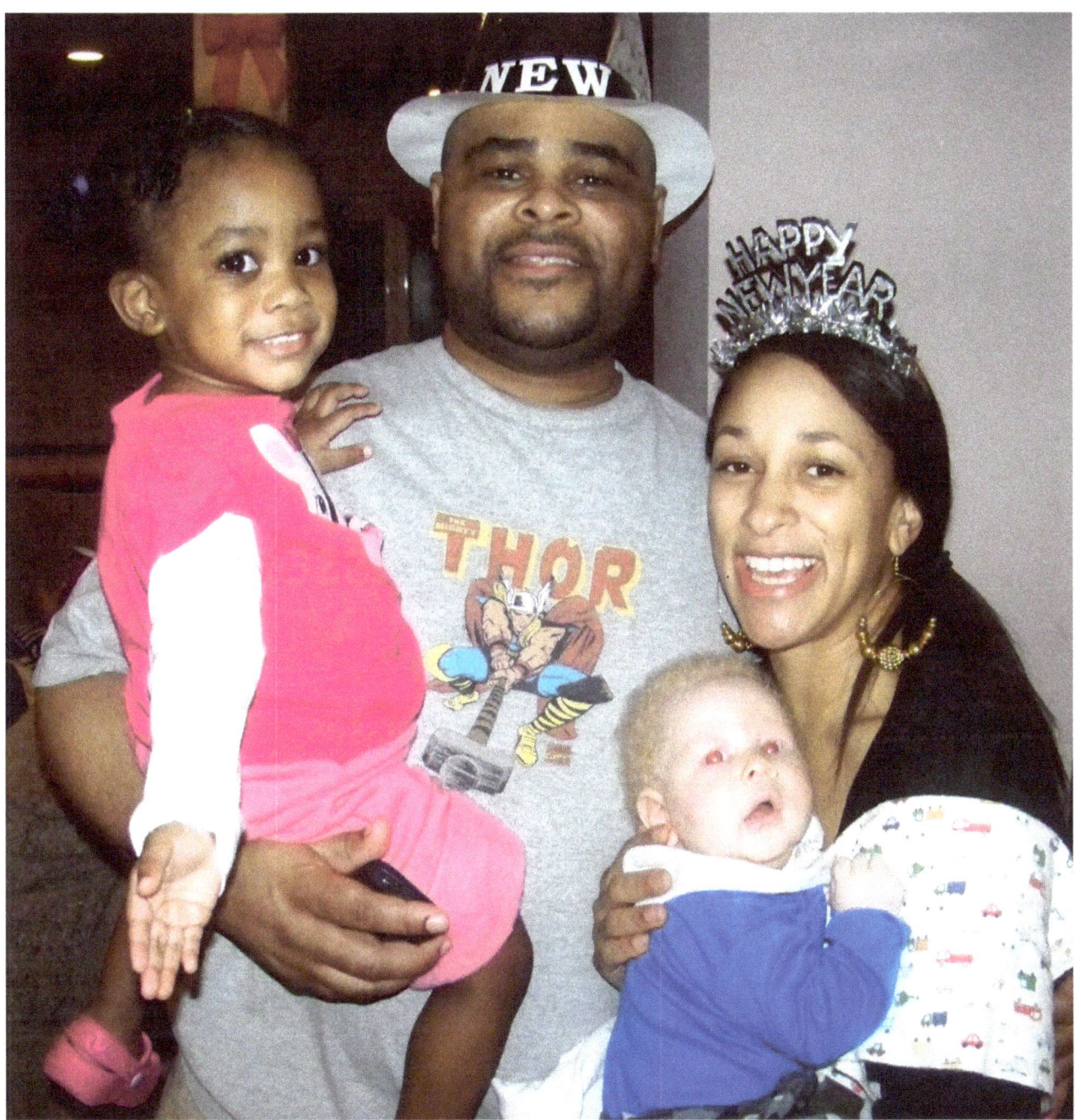

# How and Why I Protect My Skin

# My Cool Sunglasses

My super cool sunglasses protect my eyes from bright lights, especially the sun!

People with Albinism do not have color on their iris to help block the sunshine. I wear sunglasses to protect my eyes from sunlight and some indoor lighting that may be too bright.

People without Albinism have built-in sunglasses (color on their iris) to help block the sunshine.

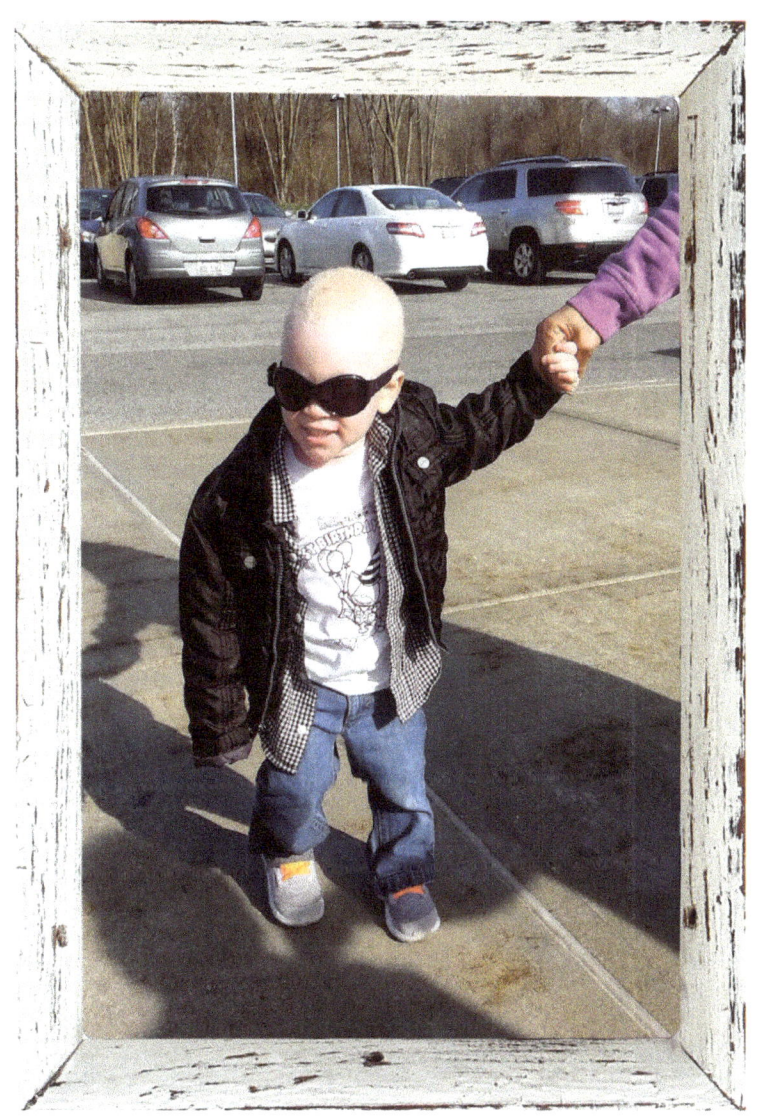

# My Hats

I wear hats outdoors to protect my head, eyes, and neck from the sun's rays. Bucket hats are my favorite!

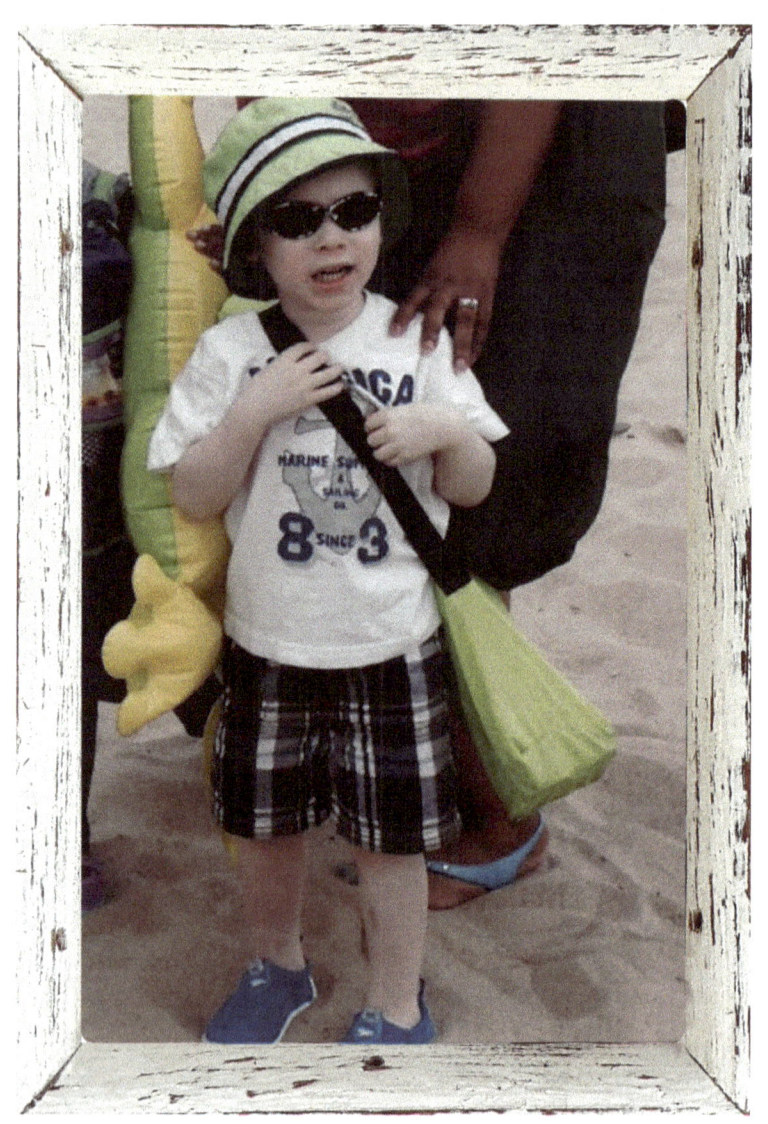

# My Sunblock

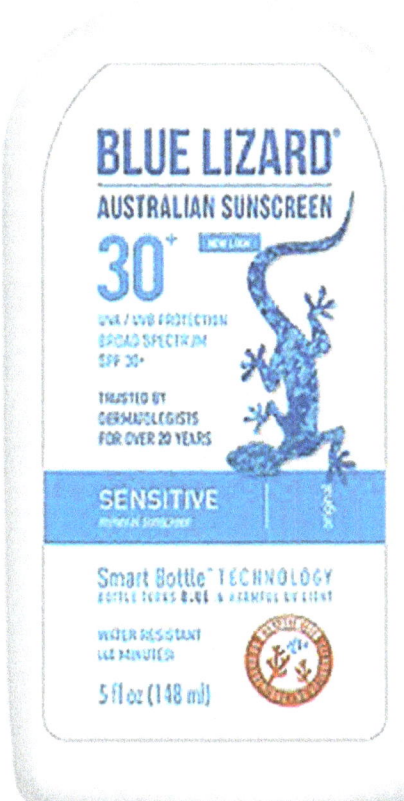

I use sunblock on my skin every day. It helps protect my skin from the sun's ultraviolet rays. Are you protecting your skin?

The FDA recommends everyone use sunblock to prevent the possibility of skin cancer.

# My Eyes

I CAN see! My eyes appear to be blue or gray. I have nystagmus (ny-stag-mus), which makes my eyes move from side to side. I hold things close to see better. You have HD vision and mine is low definition, kind of like your TV. I also have a 'nullpoint', I tilt my head to focus on one thing.

Some PWA's may or may not be able drive.

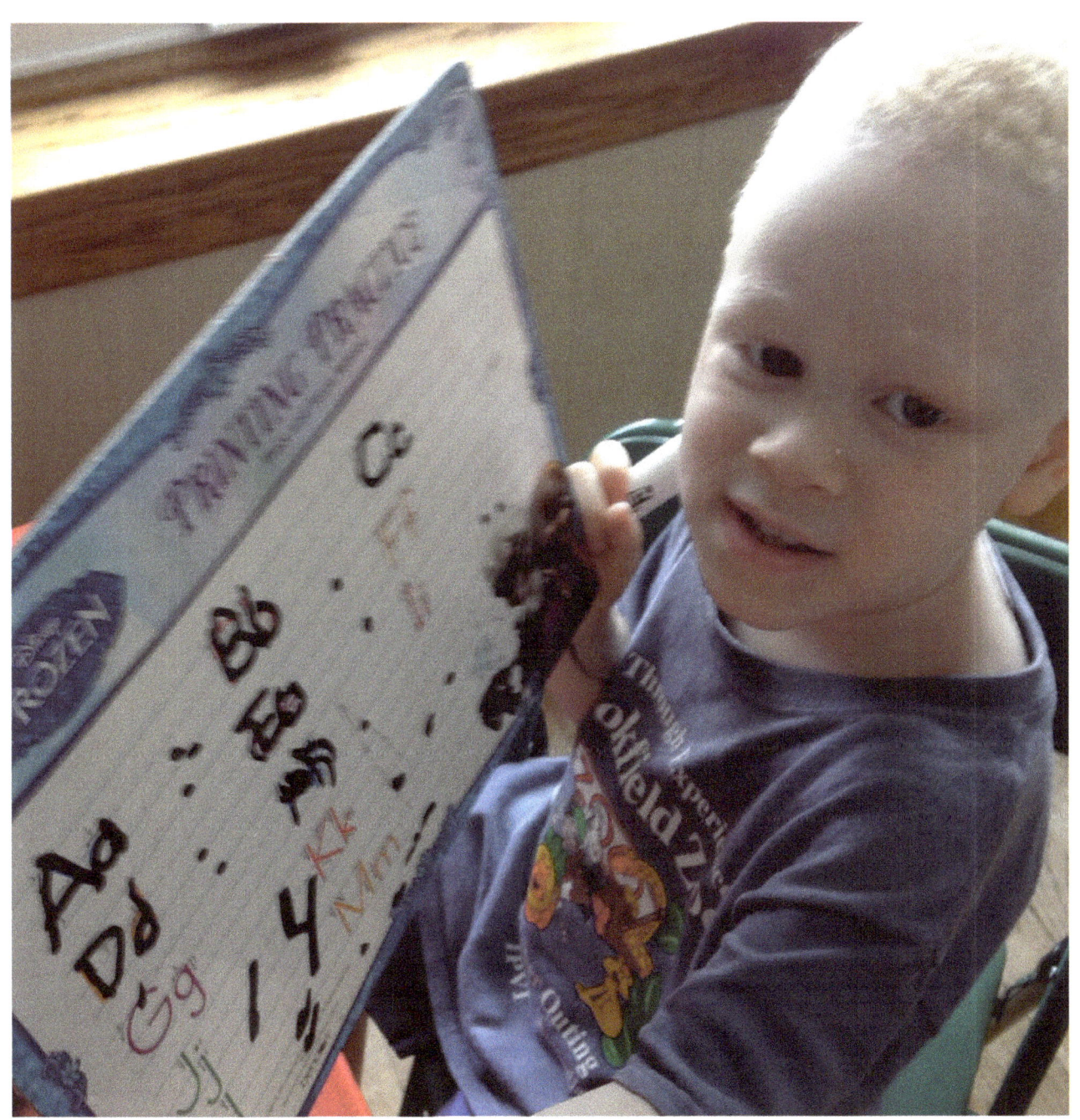

# My Super Sister!

Every superhero has a *"Team-up"*. Mine is my six year-old sister, Korryn. She is my best friend and I love her to pieces. Korryn does not have albinism, but she is extra special too!

*\*According to NOAH, "In the U.S., approximately one in 18,000 to 20,000 people has some type of albinism. In other parts of the world, the occurrence can be as high as one in 3,000".*
https://www.albinism.org/information-bulletin-what-is-albinism/

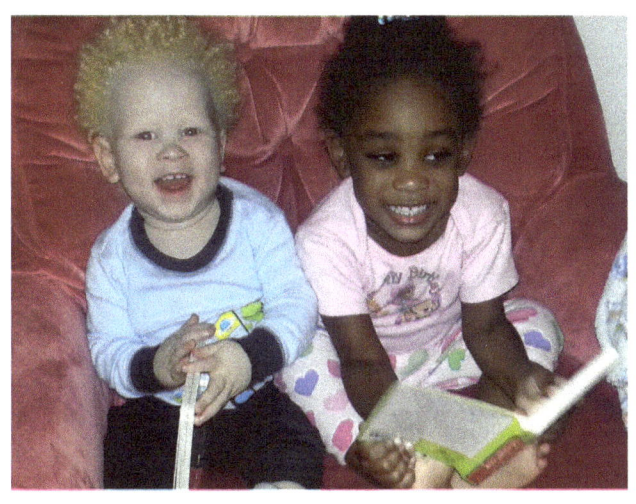 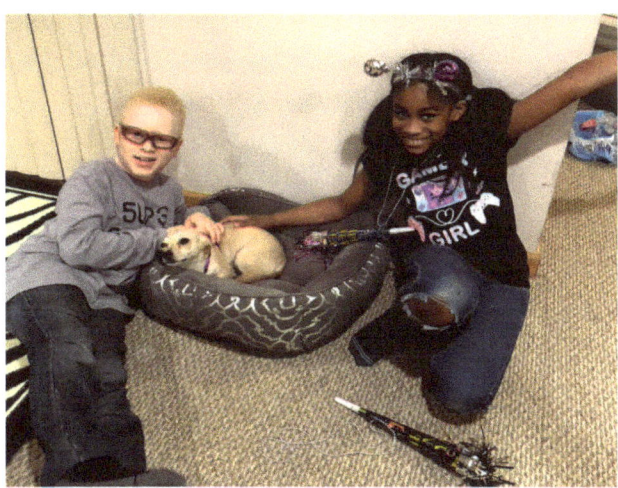
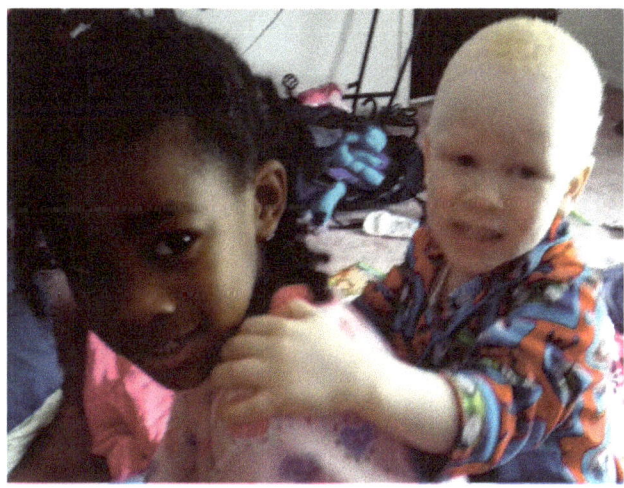 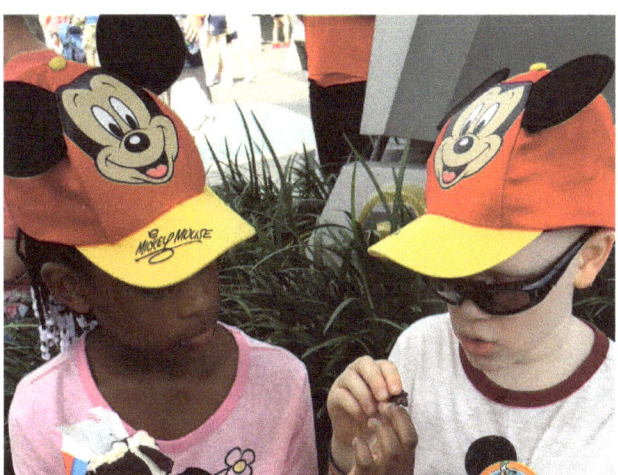

# How School Works for Me

I have a vision itinerant (teacher) who makes seeing my school work much easier.

She trains me on how to use my super tools like the cool ones on the next page.

# MY SUPER TOOLS

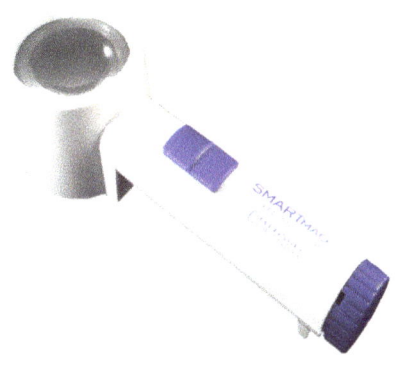

Magnifier - SuperWord Illuminator

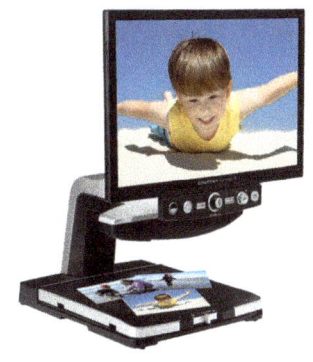

SuperCCTV allows me to see my work and other images closer

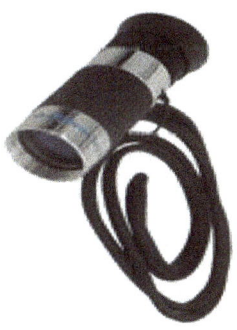

Monocular/Telescope Focus SuperSizer

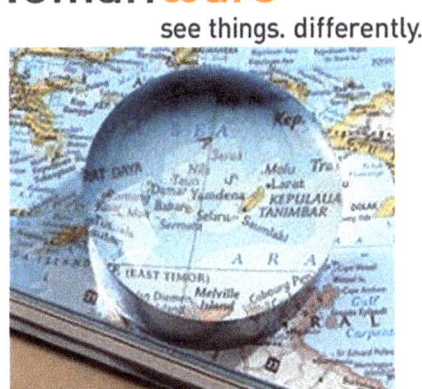

Dome MagnifiercDual Super Word/Imager SuperSizer

# NOAH

My family and I belong to an organization called **NOAH**. It offers a lot of resources for me and my family. It is also a way for me to connect with other Super PWA's!

*"NOAH's mission is to act as a conduit for accurate and authoritative information about all aspects of living with albinism and to provide a place where people with albinism and their families in the U.S. and Canada can find acceptance, support, and fellowship."
https://www.albinism.org/about-noah/

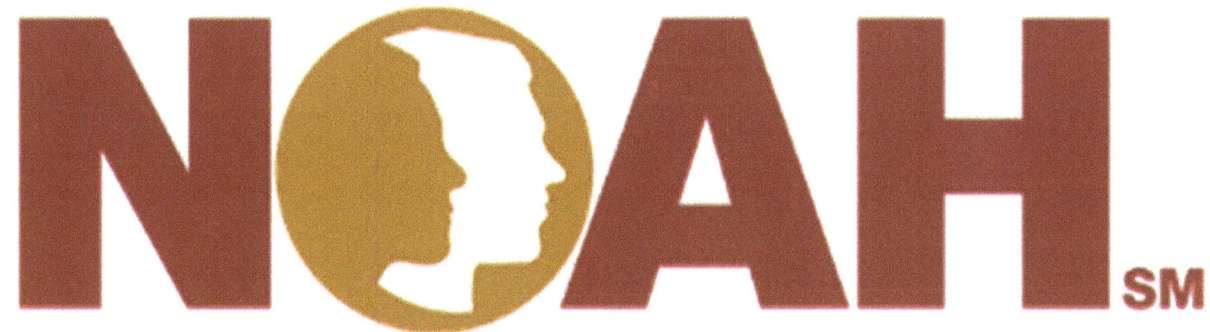

# For more information on albinism, visit www.albinism.org

NOAH was instrumental in helping me get casted for a video shoot. Here are some photos with my *"Team-Up"* for Castlecomer's video titled "All of the Noise".

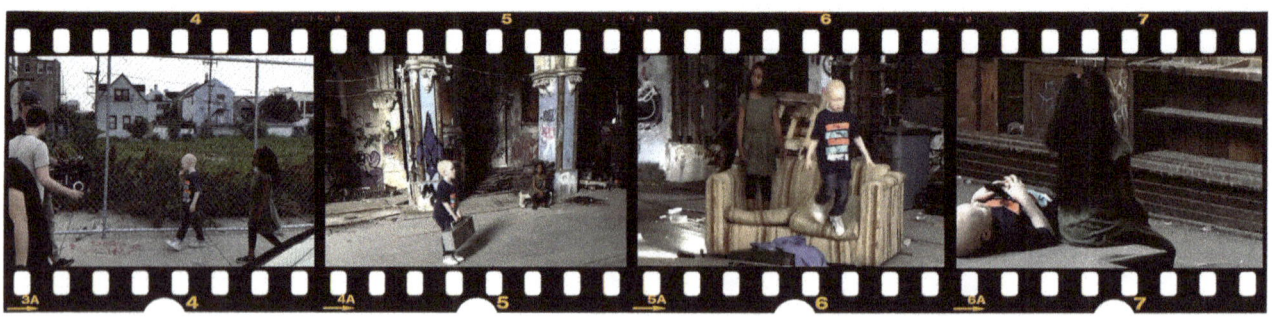

# Here are friends I met through NOAH, who dare to be different, successful, and a trailblazer for superheroes like me.

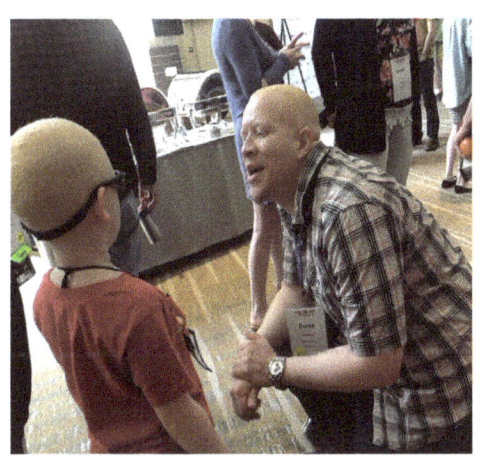

## Donte' Mickens

Financial Analyst, Paralympian for Goalball, and Board Chair for NOAH

https://www.teamusa.org/para-goalball/athletes/Donte-Mickens

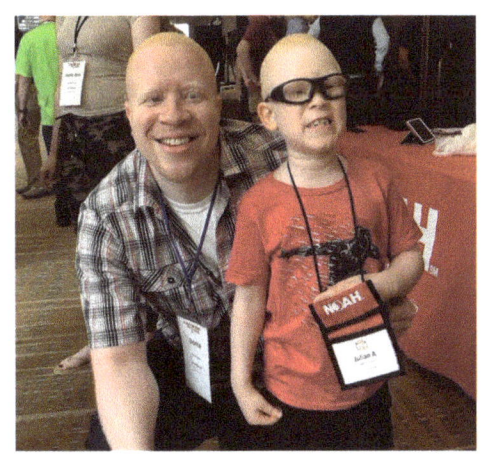

## Torey Alford
**Technical Lead for BlackSky**
Which is a geospatial service that takes satellite photos of Earth. Board Chair for NOAH, the first person with albinism to bicycle across the United States from Yorktown, VA to San Francisco, CA., an avid rock climber, cyclist, skier, hiker ... all around outdoor enthusiast!

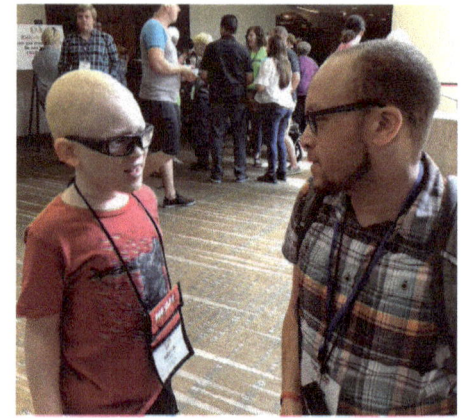

## Mike McGowan
**Executive Director of NOAH**

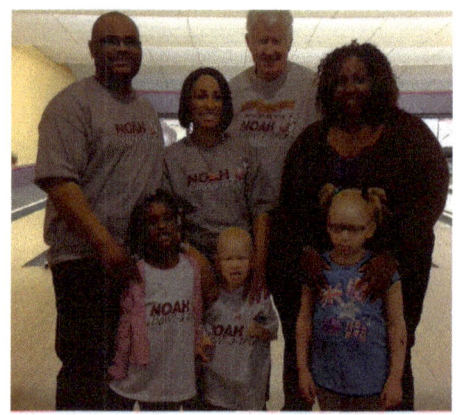

## Charli and Joshie
**My First Friends with Albinism**

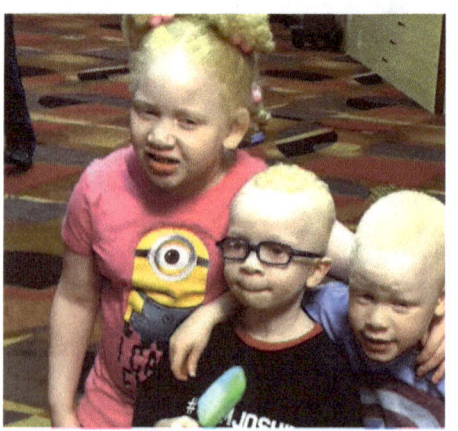

# I LOVE ME!

Overall, I am an average four year-old boy living with albinism who may look different. I still like to have fun, learn, laugh, and love just like YOU! See, it is ok to be different because in some ways we are all the same.

Here are a few of
my favorite things I like to do. Find
one that you like to do ?

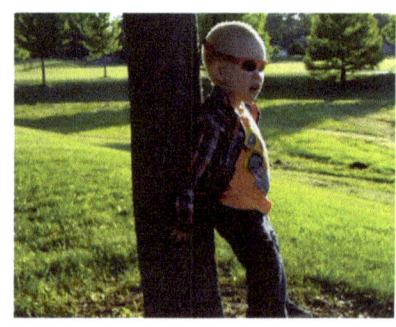 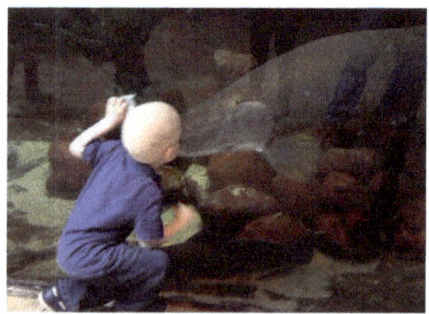 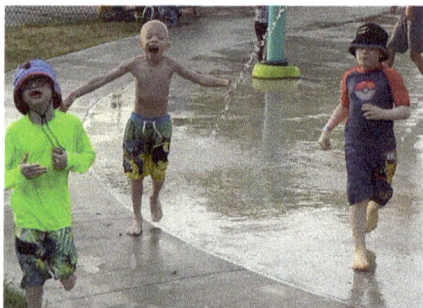

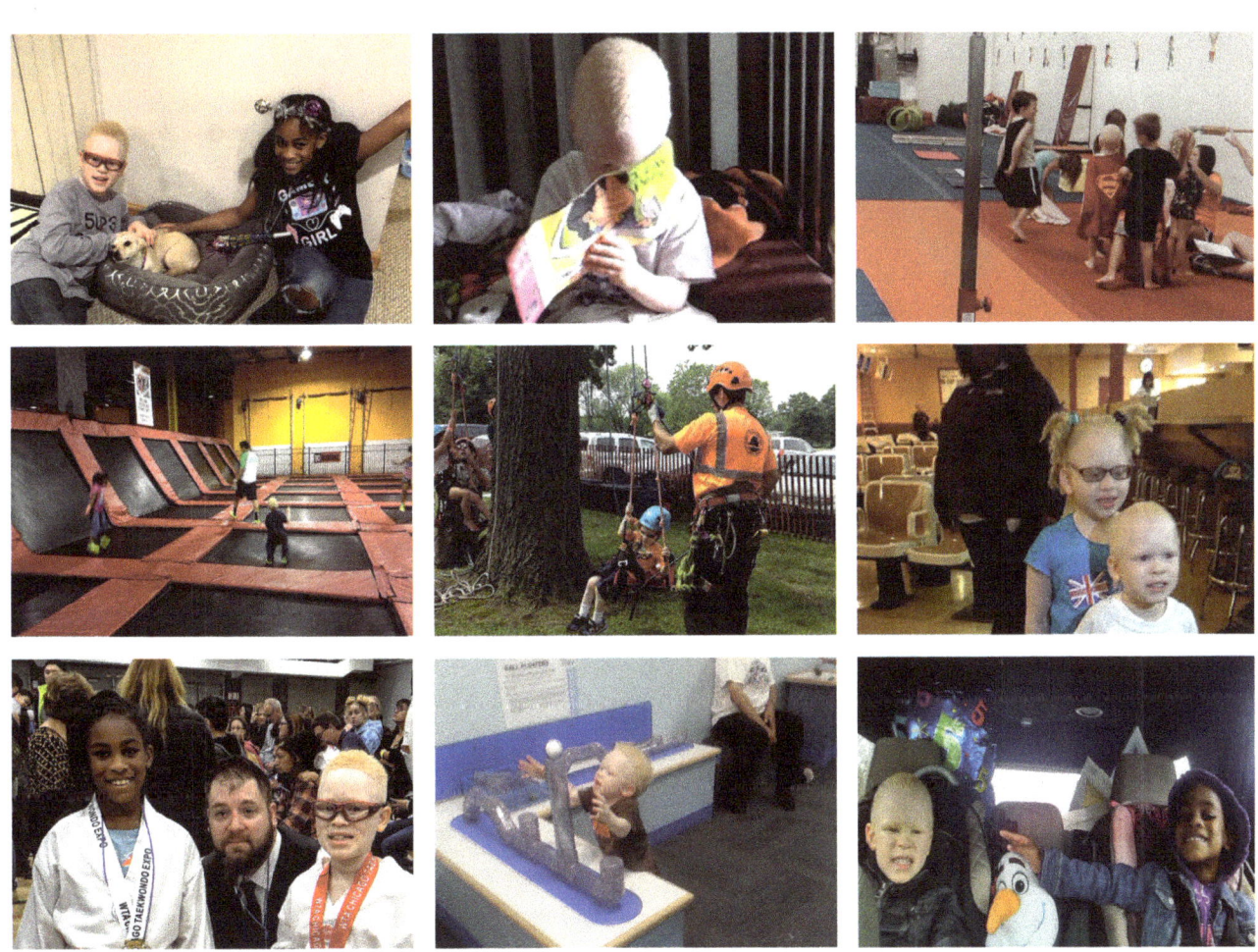

Thank you for taking this life journey of superhero JAK and his supertools. Stay tuned for the adventures of...

RESOURCES
WWW.ALBINISM.ORG (NOAH)
WWW.KIDSHEALTH.ORG

Draw or write a story about **YOUR** hero using the following pages...

www.ingramcontent.com/pod-product-compliance
Lightning Source LLC
Chambersburg PA
CBHW061149010526
44118CB00026B/2921